THE 14-DAY SCARSDALE DIET MEAL PLAN

A Nutritional Blueprint for Rapid Weight Loss, Enhanced Metabolism and Enjoy Delicious Low-Carbohydrate, High Protein Recipes

Joe Miller, RD

Copyright Page

Copyright © 2024 Joe Miller, RD

Table of Contents

INTRODUCTION

For those looking to lose weight, the Scarsdale Diet is a well-planned and rigorous program that uses calorie restriction and the intentional addition of high-protein foods to great effect. The innovative and groundbreaking Scarsdale Diet Plan, developed by the famous American cardiologist Dr. Herman Tarnower, has become famous for its easy and systematic way to lose weight. Tarnower is justifiably called the "Scarsdale Diet Doctor."

While most specialists in the field recommend cutting carbs drastically to lose weight quickly, the

Scarsdale Diet boldly goes against this grain. Proposing a dietary philosophy that advocates for a food ratio of 30% carbs, 23% fats, and the remaining amount devoted to protein, the diet highlights the intentional matching of certain meals. By combining these ingredients in such a measured way, you may create meals that are so well-planned that you can have a calorie deficit of almost 1000 each day.

In its essence, the Scarsdale Diet is more than just a weight loss program; it is an approach to overall wellbeing. The program's goals include promoting quick weight loss and protecting against several health issues, such as diabetes, high blood pressure, and heart disease. Even if you don't lose weight, the diet still has a plethora of other advantages, such as more energy, better digestion, and better sleep. Essentially, the Scarsdale Diet is a model of holistic health, with each carefully chosen food item acting as a lynchpin in the quest for peak physical and mental performance.

CHAPTER 1
Scarsdale Diet Overview

In the 1970s, the Scarsdale Diet became well-known as an easy way to lose weight. This weight loss program was developed by cardiologist Dr. Herman Tarnower and centers on cutting calories drastically while maintaining a certain ratio of fat, carbs, and protein.

An essential component of the Scarsdale Diet is a low-carb, high-protein eating plan that is intended to initiate weight reduction in a short period of time. This program is perfect for people who need to lose weight fast for a particular occasion or who want to start a long-term weight reduction journey because the main objective is to obtain results within two weeks.

Lean meats, such as fish and chicken, plus a variety of fruits and vegetables make up the bulk of the Scarsdale Diet's somewhat strict daily meal. Minimal carbs with an emphasis on complex, fiber-rich foods. A lot of lipids, high-fat dairy products, and added sweets are off-limits on this diet.

The Scarsdale Diet's "Keep Trim" meals are a significant component that continue to be followed beyond the first two weeks of the program. Because they provide a more healthy and long-term eating plan, these meals help people keep the weight off.

Although the Scarsdale Diet has received rave reviews for its quick weight reduction effects, it is crucial to proceed with caution when following it. Some people think the diet is too restrictive and might cause dietary shortages. They also think it will be hard to follow for a long time. Anyone with preexisting health concerns should talk to their doctor before beginning any new diet program.

The Scarsdale Diet is a regimented way to lose weight quickly in a controlled environment. It is important to weigh the benefits against any risks and talk to a doctor to make sure it fits with your specific health objectives and circumstances, even though it could work for the short term.

Historical Background

Dr. Herman Tarnower's high-protein, low-carbohydrate Scarsdale Diet was a popular weight control program in the 1970s. The principal objective of the diet, developed by Dr. Tarnower, a cardiologist situated in Scarsdale, New York, was to assist patients in losing weight and improving their general health. Thanks to its straightforward approach and guaranteed fast weight reduction results, the program went viral in no time.

The Scarsdale Diet is based on the principle of consuming a moderate amount of protein, carbs, and fats, with an emphasis on lean protein. In order to lose weight effectively, the strategy recommends limiting caloric intake each day. Dr. Tarnower's strategy was based on the idea that substantial weight loss might be achieved by cutting calories while keeping nutrients balanced.

Among the many things that set the Scarsdale Diet apart is its rigid menu, which details exactly what people should consume for two weeks. Among the many items on the menu are lean meats, fresh produce, and minimal carbs. The diet minimizes snacking in between meals and emphasizes portion management. Some who advocated for the diet said that it was easier to stick to because of how regimented it was.

Although many people have found success on the Scarsdale Diet, not all nutritionists and doctors are on board with it. Some have voiced worries that the diet might not be able to provide enough of certain nutrients in the long run. Problems with sticking to the suggested eating habits could also arise if the meal plan's strict structure doesn't work for everyone.

Unfortunately, Dr. Herman Tarnower's life became entangled in scandal after his longtime lover, Jean Harris, tragically murdered him in 1980. The scandal ended the life of the Scarsdale

Diet's originator in a shocking and sad way. Those looking for a regimented way to lose weight, however, have continued to follow the program in its many forms and variants.

When it first came out, the Scarsdale Diet changed the face of nutrition and weight loss forever. As the area of nutrition has progressed via new trends and research, its historical importance rests in the fact that it was an early advocate for a regimented, calorie-controlled diet.

Objectives and Intentions

Designed by Dr. Herman Tarnower, the Scarsdale Diet promotes health and weight loss in a systematic and efficient manner. Rapid weight reduction is a key goal of this diet, which employs a targeted combination of dietary restrictions and calorie counting to do just that. The goal is to speed up the metabolism and promote fat burning by adhering to a balanced, low-calorie eating plan.

Encouraging individuals to make conscious and nutritious eating choices is another important purpose of the Scarsdale Diet, which is to encourage a better lifestyle. Foods that are heavy in calories and processed are discouraged on this diet, which instead promotes a diet rich in fresh produce and lean meats. In addition to helping with weight reduction, this method tries to encourage the kind of habits that will keep you healthy in the long run.

The Scarsdale Diet focuses on the mental side of food consumption in addition to weight loss. The goal of offering a simple and easy-to-follow meal plan is to help people keep to the rules by reducing choice fatigue. This methodical strategy encourages self-control and discipline in relation to food intake.

Teaching people how to regulate their portions and eat mindfully is another goal of the Scarsdale Diet. The diet aims to provide a realistic and lasting weight reduction plan that people may follow by stressing the need of moderation and balance. With this educational component, we hope to encourage people to be active participants in their own healthcare and to make educated decisions about what they eat.

The goals of the Scarsdale Diet are to help people lose weight quickly, eat healthily, deal with the emotional and mental components of food, and learn how to live a healthy lifestyle. The goal of the diet is to promote health and weight loss in a comprehensive way by combining these objectives.

CHAPTER 2
Understanding the Science Behind the Scarsdale Diet

The goal of this weight reduction regimen is to facilitate rapid weight loss by use of a combination of calorie restriction and dietary restriction.

Reducing caloric intake is fundamental to the Scarsdale Diet. The recommended daily consumption of calories is 1,000 to 1,100, which is far lower than the usual caloric intake of most people. It is thought that by causing the body to use its stored fat for energy, this calorie deficit causes weight reduction to occur rapidly.

Following the diet's prescribed meal plan is essential; it stresses the need of eating enough of fruits and vegetables, lean meats, and low-fat or no-fat dairy products. The objective is to get into ketosis, when your body uses fat instead of carbs for fuel, when you're not getting enough carbs. This change in metabolism is believed to have a role in the diet's ability to promote weight reduction.

Consumption of foods high in protein is central to the Scarsdale Diet. The digestion and processing of protein requires more energy than other macronutrients because of its increased thermic impact. In addition to aiding weight reduction by keeping muscle mass intact, this may also help you feel full for longer. Fruits and vegetables are promoted as part of the diet because of the many health benefits they provide, including vitamins, minerals, and fiber.

The Scarsdale Diet has its detractors who worry about its long-term viability due to the extreme calorie restriction and restricted food options it imposes. Rapid weight reduction on low-calorie diets may be due to water weight loss as well as muscle mass loss, not only fat.

People thinking about going on the Scarsdale Diet or any other kind of restrictive diet should talk to their doctor beforehand. Prior to beginning a weight reduction program, one should give serious thought to their own health concerns, dietary requirements, and the plan's long-term viability. For long-term health and wellness, it's best to eat properly and exercise regularly, not only for the short-term effects that the Scarsdale Diet may provide.

Diet Principles of Scarsdale Diet

One well-known and organized method of losing weight is the Scarsdale Diet, which stresses cutting calories while maintaining a healthy nutritional balance. The goal of this diet is to help people lose weight quickly by limiting their caloric intake and sticking to a certain meal combination. Reducing carbohydrate consumption and increasing protein-rich food consumption is central to the Scarsdale Diet.

Meals on this diet are meticulously prepared to incorporate a range of lean proteins such chicken, fish, and lean cuts of meat, with plenty of veggies. By cutting back on calorie-heavy carbs and fats, you can keep your calorie deficit in check. In addition to helping with weight reduction, this also makes sure that your body gets all the nutrients it needs to be healthy.

The Scarsdale Diet also stresses the need of controlling one's portion sizes. People may help the diet work better by managing their portion sizes and measuring out exactly how many calories they eat. This method offers a long-term solution to the problem of obesity since it controls blood sugar levels and stops people from eating too much.

One of the Scarsdale Diet's tenets is "maintaining momentum." To initiate weight reduction, this method entails sticking to the eating regimen religiously for a set amount of time, often two weeks. After this first stage, many go on to a maintenance plan that is more accommodating, letting them eat more of what they want but still focusing on portion control and good eating habits.

Fruits, especially those low in sugar, are highly recommended by the Scarsdale Diet because of the many vitamins and minerals they contain. In addition to helping with weight reduction, this also encourages a healthy, balanced diet.

The Scarsdale Diet advocates a well-rounded diet that includes nutrient-dense meals, moderate carbohydrate intake, portion management, and overall good health. The diet's goal is to help people lose weight in a healthy way, therefore it starts off by being strict but eventually becomes more accommodating as long as they stick to the good eating habits. Prior to making substantial dietary adjustments, it is recommended to get advice from a healthcare practitioner, as is the case with any diet plan.

Mechanism of Scarsdale Diet

Fundamental to the Scarsdale Diet is the idea of calorie restriction, with an emphasis on a certain macronutrient ratio.

Consumption of a restricted caloric intake is central to the Scarsdale Diet. The calorie consumption is deliberately maintained low, usually between 1,000 and 1,200 calories per day. By forcing the body to use its fat stores for energy, this calorie restriction plan aims to induce weight reduction.

An important part of the Scarsdale Diet's mechanism is the allocation of macronutrients. According to the diet plan, protein should make up around 43% of calories, carbs 34.5 %, and fat 22.5 %. With this low-carb, high-protein strategy, you can train your body to burn fat for energy instead of carbs, which will keep you from eating too much and from being too hungry.

In order to help you maintain your muscle mass while you lose weight, the Scarsdale Diet recommends eating lean protein sources including chicken, fish, and low-fat dairy. The goal of reducing carbohydrate consumption is to maintain a steady energy balance by reducing insulin resistance and the likelihood of dangerous blood sugar rises.

The Scarsdale Diet is also known for its regimented eating schedule, which usually calls for three square meals a day with predetermined ingredient combinations. Vegetables, fruits, and lean meats are all part of the regimen, whereas processed and high-calorie items are off limits.

It's worth noting that the Scarsdale Diet can provide quick weight reduction in the beginning, but its detractors say it won't work in the long run. Meeting nutritional needs may be difficult on this diet, and sticking to it for long periods of time may be even more of a difficulty due to its lack of variety.

The Scarsdale Diet works by limiting calories, following a certain macronutrient ratio, and having a planned meal schedule. While this diet may help you lose weight quickly, it has certain drawbacks that you should know about and talk to your doctor about before you make any major changes to your eating habits.

Advantages and Drawbacks of Scarsdale Diet

The fact that it is easy to understand and implement is a major plus when it comes to losing weight. A calorie deficit, which the diet encourages with its focus on protein and minimal carbs, can speed up the weight reduction process. Those looking for a straightforward diet, free of complicated computations and time-consuming meal preparation, would like its simplicity.

Additionally, the Scarsdale Diet provides a wide range of foods to choose from, which helps keep people from getting bored and makes the diet more manageable in the long run. A balanced nutritional profile is achieved by including lean proteins, fruits, and vegetables, which prevent the complete neglect of key elements.

The Scarsdale Diet, however, is not without its flaws. The fact that it restricts some food categories and could not offer a balanced nutritional answer in the long run is a major worry. While cutting out carbohydrates could cause you to lose weight quickly at first, it could also cause you to lose nutrients and have energy dumps later on. In addition, some people may find it difficult to follow the rules, which raises the possibility that they may quit the diet.

Another negative aspect of the Scarsdale Diet is that it does not prioritize physical activity. Regular physical exercise to enhance general health and fitness should ideally be a part of any comprehensive weight reduction plan, even when the diet mostly focuses on nutritional adjustments. The lack of an organized exercise component in the diet might make it less efficient in helping people lose weight and stay healthy after the early phases.

The Scarsdale Diet provides a variety of foods to choose from and clear instructions for losing weight in an easy and approachable way. Overall, its efficacy and influence on nutritional balance are questionable due to its restrictive character and possible inadequacy of long-term maintenance. A balanced and long-term strategy for weight control is essential, so anybody thinking about trying this diet should think carefully about the pros and downsides.

CHAPTER 3
Initiating the Journey on the of Scarsdale Diet

Starting the Scarsdale Diet feels like stepping into a life-altering adventure towards a healthier and more vibrant me. I want to make healthy adjustments to my lifestyle and put my health first, therefore I've decided to follow this diet plan.

As I explore the Scarsdale Diet more, I am amazed by its supposed ability to help people lose weight rapidly and effectively. The organized meal plan gives me a clear road map for my daily nutrition, and the focus on a low-carb, high-protein strategy sounds good.

Starting a new diet program is always an adventure, but it can also be a bit of a struggle. Because it emphasizes eating plenty of fresh produce, lean meats, and healthy fats, the Scarsdale Diet should be delicious. My taste senses may take some time to adjust to this new eating plan, but I'm excited to find new ways to enjoy every meal.

The Scarsdale Diet stresses the importance of preparation, so I make sure to include fresh vegetables, lean meats, and other necessities on my shopping lists. Breakfast, lunch, supper, and snacks are all part of the well-organized meal plan, which gives me direction and aids in resisting temptation.

I understand that making a drastic adjustment to one's eating habits calls for self-control and dedication. Nevertheless, what keeps me going is reading about people's success stories and testimonies about the Scarsdale Diet. Their stories of success—increased energy, visible weight reduction, and great experiences—motivate me to keep going.

The need for moderation and balance is something I am conscious of, even as I am enthusiastic about the likely advantages. I like that the Scarsdale Diet stresses the need of making a change to a more sustainable, long-term strategy in order to keep the weight off.

CHAPTER 4

The Scarsdale Diet Meal Blueprint

The main goal of the Scarsdale Diet is to help people lose weight quickly. It also aims to improve health by lowering the risk of heart disease, high blood pressure, and diabetes. Other benefits include more energy, better digestion, and improved sleep.

This diet focuses on eating fewer calories, limiting carbs and fats, and emphasizing lean protein, fruits, and vegetables. It is low in sodium and high

The 14-Day Scarsdale Diet Meal Plan 32

in fiber, with about 43% of calories from protein, 22.5% from fat, and 34.5% from carbs. The daily calorie intake is around 1,000 calories.

While the limited food choices can seem boring, getting creative with your meals can make the diet enjoyable and effective. Here are some recipe ideas to spice up your meal plan, which can be paired with fat-burning supplements available online.

The Scarsdale Diet is a two-week plan with specific daily food requirements. The second week is the same as the first. After these two weeks, you can add more foods for the next two weeks. Using Scarsdale Diet recipes can keep you motivated and help improve your results. Adding superfoods and taking care of your mental health can also help.

To stick to the diet, follow these rules: eat only the assigned foods each day, avoid alcohol, and if you need a snack, stick to carrots or celery (as much as you want). Allowed drinks are coffee, tea, club soda, diet sodas, and water, with only artificial sweeteners and lemon.

Permitted Foods

Foods you can eat on the Scarsdale Diet include:

Meat, Poultry, and Seafood: Chicken, turkey, beef, lamb, steak, fish, and shellfish.

Drinks: Black coffee, tea, and water.

Cheese: Low-fat varieties like cottage cheese.

Eggs: Prepared without oil or other fats.

Cold Cuts: Various deli meats.

Vegetables: Non-starchy vegetables like carrots and celery.

Low-Fat Dairy: 2% milk, low-fat cheeses, and low-fat yogurt.

Fruits: Grapefruit is emphasized, but all fruits are allowed.

Seasonings: Most herbs and spices.

Beverages: Unsweetened black coffee, tea, zero-calorie diet soda, and water.

Protein Bread: Made of soy flour, whole wheat flour, and gluten flour, commonly mentioned in the diet book and available in grocery stores in the 1970s.

Prohibited Foods

The Scarsdale Diet restricts many food groups, including some that are generally considered healthy, without explaining why. The restricted foods are:

Starchy Vegetables: Eggplant, sweet potatoes, white potatoes, beets, butternut squash, turnips, peas.

Legumes: Black beans, kidney beans, chickpeas, lentils.

Full-Fat Dairy: Whole milk, yogurt, and fatty cheeses like cheddar, Parmesan, and Swiss.

Fats and Oils: All oils, butter, ghee, mayonnaise, and salad dressings.

Wheat and Grains: Bread, breakfast cereals, pasta, sandwiches, wraps.

Nuts and Seeds: All nuts and seeds except walnuts and pecans (in limited amounts).

Processed Meats: Bacon, chorizo, calamari, ham, sausages, corned beef.

Junk Foods: French fries, donuts, cookies, cakes, fast foods.

Sweets and Desserts: All sweets and desserts, including chocolate.

Processed Foods: Fast food, frozen food, potato chips, premade dinners, etc.

Sugar-Sweetened Beverages: Most fruit juices, sugary sodas, tea and coffee with added sugar, sports drinks.

Avocados

Alcohol

CHAPTER 5
HIGH PROTEIN, LOW-CALORIE
BREAKFAST RECIPES

Jimmbo's Garlic Knots

Ingredients You Need

1 (10 ounce) can refrigerated pizza crust dough

⅓ cup olive oil

6 tablespoons finely chopped fresh garlic

5 tablespoons grated Parmesan cheese

3 tablespoons chopped fresh parsley

1 teaspoon crushed red pepper

1 teaspoon salt

How to Make

Preheat the oven to 450 degrees F (230 degrees C).

Roll out pizza dough to form a 10x16-inch sheet of dough. Cut sheet into 3/4-inch parallel strips. Then cut these strips in half, making about 24 pieces. Tie each strip into a knot and place them close together on a greased pan.

Bake in the preheated oven until golden brown.

Immediately transfer hot knots to a large bowl and drizzle with olive oil. Sprinkle with garlic, cheese, parsley, red pepper, and salt. Toss well and serve.

Cottage Cheese Breakfast Bowl

Ingredients You Need

2 slices bacon, chopped

2 medium fresh mushrooms, chopped

1 tablespoon minced green onions (including green tops)

salt and ground black pepper to taste

2 eggs, lightly beaten

½ cup cottage cheese

How to Make

Cook bacon in a small nonstick skillet over medium heat until browned, 4 to 5 minutes. Transfer bacon to a paper towel-lined bowl, reserving bacon grease in a small bowl.

Return skillet to medium-high heat and add 1 teaspoon reserved bacon grease. Cook mushrooms and green onions until lightly browned, 3 to 4 minutes. Season with salt and pepper. Transfer to a small bowl and keep warm.

Return skillet to medium-high heat and add 1 teaspoon reserved bacon grease. Add eggs and scramble until cooked through, 2 to 3 minutes. Season with salt and pepper. Remove from heat and keep warm.

Place cottage cheese into a microwave-safe bowl. Heat on 50% power for 60 to 90 seconds, or until warm, stirring halfway through. Drain any liquid that has been released and transfer cottage cheese into one side of a single-serving bowl. Place scrambled eggs into the other side of the bowl. Top with mushroom mixture and bacon. Serve immediately.

Please Note

If you do not have enough bacon grease to make 2 teaspoons, use butter or oil to make up the difference.

Fluffy Keto Pancakes

Ingredients You Need

1 cup almond flour

¼ cup coconut flour

2 tablespoons low-calorie natural sweetener (such as Swerve®)

1 teaspoon salt

1 teaspoon baking powder

½ teaspoon ground cinnamon (Optional)

6 eggs, at room temperature

¼ cup heavy whipping cream, at room temperature

2 tablespoons butter, melted

1 teaspoon vanilla extract

How to Make

Mix almond flour, coconut flour, sweetener, salt, baking powder, and cinnamon together in a bowl. Whisk in eggs, heavy cream, butter, and vanilla extract slowly until batter is just blended.

Heat a lightly oiled griddle over medium-high heat. Drop batter by large spoonfuls onto the griddle and cook until bubbles form and the edges are dry, 3 to 4 minutes. Flip and cook until browned on the other side, 2 to 3 minutes. Repeat with remaining batter.

Low-Carb Lemon Poppy Seed Muffins

Ingredients You Need

⅓ cup low-calorie natural sweetener (such as Swerve®)

¼ cup almond flour

¼ cup coconut flour

1 tablespoon poppy seeds

1 lemon, zested

½ teaspoon baking powder

½ teaspoon salt

¼ teaspoon xanthan gum (Optional)

3 large eggs

3 tablespoons butter

2 tablespoons sour cream

½ teaspoon vanilla extract

2 tablespoons heavy whipping cream, or more to taste

How to Make

Preheat the oven to 350 degrees F (175 degrees C). Grease a muffin tin or line with paper muffin liners.

Mix sweetener, almond flour, coconut flour, poppy seeds, lemon zest, baking powder, salt, and xanthan gum together in a bowl.

Beat eggs in a bowl with an electric mixer on high speed until fluffy, about 2 minutes. Beat in butter, sour cream, and vanilla. Add sweetener mixture.

Stir in cream slowly until batter is thick and smooth. Pour into the prepared muffin tin.

Bake in the preheated oven until tops are golden, 15 to 20 minutes.

Please Note

Xanthan gum helps improve texture but is not vital to the recipe.

You will need 1 to 4 tablespoons heavy cream depending on the size of the eggs used.

Coconut oil can be substituted for the butter if desired.

Cauliflower Hash Browns

Ingredients You Need

3 cups grated cauliflower

1 cup shredded Cheddar cheese

1 large egg

¼ cup real bacon bits

1 tablespoon diced chives

½ teaspoon salt

⅛ teaspoon ground black pepper

1 pinch cayenne pepper (Optional)

cooking spray

How to Make

Preheat the oven to 400 degrees F (200 degrees C).

Place grated cauliflower in a microwave-safe bowl. Cook on high for 2 minutes. Let cool for 5 minutes.

Wring cauliflower in a clean dish towel, squeezing out as much moisture as possible. Transfer cauliflower to a large mixing bowl. Add Cheddar cheese, egg, bacon bits, chives, salt, pepper, and cayenne. Mix well.

Spray a large baking sheet with cooking spray. Divide cauliflower mixture into 6 equal portions, making sure to leave space between each one. Flatten with your hands and shape into ovals.

Bake in the preheated oven until browned, about 15 minutes. Turn broiler on low and broil until crispy, about 5 minutes. Let cool for 5 minutes to firm up.

Avocado Egg Bake

Ingredients You Need

2 large eggs

1 medium avocado, halved and pitted

¼ cup shredded Cheddar cheese

salt and freshly ground black pepper to taste

1 tablespoon chopped fresh parsley, or to taste (Optional)

How to Make

Preheat the oven to 425 degrees F (220 degrees C). Crack each egg into a small bowl.

Scoop some avocado flesh out from each pit cavity to make room for one egg. Place avocado halves onto a baking sheet; gently pour an egg into each cavity.

Bake in the preheated oven until eggs are cooked through, 15 to 20 minutes.

Remove from the oven and transfer to a plate. Sprinkle Cheddar cheese on top, season with salt and pepper, and garnish with parsley.

Roasted Leeks with Eggs

Ingredients You Need

2 leeks

3 green onions

2 tablespoons ghee (clarified butter), melted

½ teaspoon sea salt

¼ teaspoon ground black pepper

Avocado Vinaigrette:

1 ripe avocado, pitted, flesh scooped from skin

¾ cup light olive oil

1 lemon, juiced

¼ cup red wine vinegar

salt and ground black pepper to taste

1 teaspoon olive oil

2 eggs

¼ cup sliced almonds, toasted

⅛ teaspoon red pepper flakes

How to Make

Preheat the oven to 400 degrees F (200 degrees C).

Discard green tops and the bottom 1/2 inch of the leeks. Cut leeks in half lengthwise.

Place leeks and green onions on a sheet pan. Drizzle with ghee. Add sea salt and pepper.

Roast in the preheated oven until browned, 15 to 20 minutes.

Prepare vinaigrette by blending avocado, 3/4 cup olive oil, lemon juice, vinegar, salt, and pepper thoroughly in a food processor.

Heat 1 teaspoon oil in a skillet over medium-low heat. Crack eggs into opposite sides of the skillet and cook until whites are barely set and yolks are still runny, 2 to 3 minutes.

Remove leeks and onions from oven and top with the sunny-side up eggs. Sprinkle almonds and red pepper flakes on top. Finish with a drizzle of the avocado vinaigrette.

Editor's Note:

Nutrition data for this recipe includes the full amount of vinaigrette ingredients. The actual amount of vinaigrette consumed will vary.

Chocolate Almond Breakfast Donuts

Ingredients You Need

nonstick vegetable oil cooking spray

2 large eggs

2 tablespoons vegetable oil

3 tablespoons maple syrup

1 ¼ cups finely ground almond flour

1 ½ teaspoons baking powder

½ teaspoon kosher salt

2 tablespoons Dutch-process cocoa powder

How to Make

Preheat the oven to 375 degrees F (190 degrees C). Generously spray or brush a nonstick donut pan with cooking spray; set aside until needed.

Place eggs, vegetable oil, and maple syrup into a mixing bowl and whisk thoroughly until the mixture is emulsified, light, and a little bit foamy, 3 to 4 minutes. Add almond flour, baking powder, salt, and cocoa powder; mix everything together thoroughly with a spatula until all the almond flour is incorporated and you've achieved a very thick batter.

Transfer batter into a pastry bag, or a plastic zip-top bag with one of the corners cut off. Pipe the batter evenly into the prepared donut pan.

Dip a finger in water and smooth the tops of the batter to even out. Tap the pan on a work surface a few times to settle the batter even more.

Bake in the center of the preheated oven until a wooden skewer inserted into a donut comes out clean, 9 to 10 minutes. Let cool in the pan for 10 minutes before inverting onto a wire cooling rack. Cool completely before serving.

Please Note:

The donut pan can also be greased with soft butter.

You can use any fat of your choice instead of vegetable oil--butter, coconut oil, or extra-virgin olive oil, to name a few. You can use 1/4 teaspoon fine salt instead of kosher salt. Make sure to use high-quality Dutch-process cocoa powder. I used Bob's Red Mill(R) almond flour.

You can add a teaspoon of vanilla extract to the batter if you like.

Breakfast Burrito

Ingredients You Need

2 low carb whole wheat tortillas

4 eggs

2 tablespoons cream

1 pinch salt and white pepper

¼ teaspoon cumin powder

½ tablespoon butter

1 ½ tablespoons salsa, chunky style

2 ounces Cheddar cheese, shredded

How to Make

In a mixing bowl, beat the eggs with the cream, salsa, cumin and a pinch of salt and pepper.

In a non stick skillet over medium-high heat, melt the butter and then scramble the eggs. Just before they are set, add the cheese and fold-in until it begins to melt.

Lay the tortillas on a flat surface. Divide the eggs equally between the two and place on the bottom third of each tortilla. Fold the bottom third over tucking in. Fold in the two sides and then roll up. Serve.

Green Chile Variation

If you are not on the run and can afford a few extra carbs, then try placing these burritos into a casserole dish, spoon 2 tablespoon of 505 Green Chile Sauce over each and heat in a 350 degrees F (175 degrees C) oven for about ten minutes. Add a dollop of sour cream and serve.

Toasted Garlic Bread

Ingredients You Need

1 (1 pound) loaf Italian bread

5 tablespoons butter, softened

3 cloves garlic, crushed

2 teaspoons extra virgin olive oil

1 teaspoon dried oregano

salt and pepper to taste

1 cup shredded mozzarella cheese

How to Make

Gather all ingredients.

Set an oven rack about 6 inches from the heat source and preheat the oven's broiler. Cut loaf into ten 1-inch slices.

Mix butter, garlic, oil, oregano, salt, and pepper together in a bowl; spread butter mixture on one side of each slice of bread; arrange bread slices, butter-side up, in a single layer on a baking sheet.

Cook under the preheated broiler until slightly brown, checking frequently so they do not burn, about 3 minutes.

Top bread slices with cheese and return to broiler until cheese is slightly brown and melted, about 2 minutes.

Serve hot.

Buttery Garlic Green Beans

Ingredients You Need

1 pound fresh green beans, trimmed and snapped in half

3 tablespoons butter

3 cloves garlic, minced

⅛ teaspoon lemon-pepper seasoning, or more to taste

salt to taste

How to Make

Place green beans into a large skillet and cover with water; bring to a boil. Reduce heat to medium-low and simmer until beans just start to soften, 3 to 5 minutes.

Drain and return to the skillet. Add butter and stir until melted, 1 to 2 minutes.

Add garlic; cook until tender and fragrant, 1 to 2 minutes.

Season with lemon-pepper seasoning and salt before serving.

Garlic Croutons

Ingredients You Need

4 tablespoons butter

1 clove garlic, minced

3 (3/4 inch thick) slices French bread, cut into cubes

How to Make

Preheat the oven to 350 degrees F (175 degrees C).

Melt butter in a large skillet over medium heat. Add garlic; cook and stir until fragrant, about 1 minute. Add bread cubes and toss until coated. Transfer to a rimmed baking sheet and spread in an even layer.

Bake in the preheated oven, checking frequently to prevent burning, until crisp and dry, about 15 minutes. Let cool before using, 2 to 3 minutes.

Chicken & White Bean Soup

Ingredients You Need

2 teaspoons extra-virgin olive oil

2 leeks, white and light green parts only, cut into 1/4-inch rounds

1 tablespoon chopped fresh sage, or 1/4 teaspoon dried

2 (14 ounce) cans reduced-sodium chicken broth

2 cups water

1 (15 ounce) can cannellini beans, rinsed

1 (2 pound) roasted chicken, skin discarded, meat removed from bones and shredded (4 cups)

How to Make

Heat oil in a Dutch oven over medium-high heat. Add leeks and cook, stirring often, until soft, about 3 minutes. Stir in sage and continue cooking until aromatic, about 30 seconds. Stir in broth and water, increase heat to high, cover and bring to a boil. Add beans and chicken and cook, uncovered, stirring occasionally, until heated through, about 3 minutes. Serve hot.

Cauliflower & Kale Frittata

Ingredients You Need

2 tablespoons extra-virgin olive oil, divided

1 small onion, sliced

2 cups small cauliflower florets

¼ cup water

5 cups chopped kale

3 cloves garlic, minced

1 teaspoon chopped fresh thyme

½ teaspoon salt, divided

½ teaspoon ground pepper, divided

8 large eggs

½ teaspoon smoked paprika

½ cup crumbled goat cheese or shredded Manchego cheese

How to Make

Position a rack in upper third of oven; preheat broiler to high.

Heat 1 tablespoon oil in a large cast-iron skillet over medium heat. Add onion and cook, stirring occasionally, until starting to brown, 2 to 4 minutes. Add cauliflower and water. Cover and cook until just tender, about 6 minutes. Add kale, garlic, thyme and 1/4 teaspoon each salt and pepper; cook, stirring often, until the kale is wilted, 2 to 3 minutes.

Whisk eggs, paprika and the remaining 1/4 teaspoon salt and pepper in a large bowl. Add the vegetables to the egg mixture; gently stir to combine. Wipe the pan clean; add the remaining 1 tablespoon oil and heat over medium heat. Pour in the egg mixture and top with cheese. Cover and cook until the edges are set and the bottom is brown, 4 to 5 minutes.

Transfer the pan to the oven and broil until the top of the frittata is just cooked, 2 to 3 minutes.

Chopped Power Salad with Chicken

Ingredients You Need

¼ cup extra-virgin olive oil

3 tablespoons lemon juice

1 clove garlic, grated

½ teaspoon dried oregano

½ teaspoon sugar

¼ teaspoon salt

¼ teaspoon ground pepper

4 cups torn green-leaf lettuce

4 cups baby spinach

2 cups shredded cooked chicken

1 cup halved grape tomatoes

1 cup halved and sliced cucumber

½ cup slivered red onion

⅓ cup sliced pepperoncini

⅓ cup crumbled feta cheese

2 tablespoons toasted unsalted sunflower seeds

How to Make

Whisk oil, lemon juice, garlic, oregano, sugar, salt and pepper together in a large bowl.

Add lettuce, spinach, chicken, tomatoes, cucumber, onion and pepperoncini; toss to coat. Serve sprinkled with feta and sunflower seeds.

Vegan Burrito Bowls with Cauliflower Rice

Ingredients You Need

1 recipe Tofu Crumbles

1 (12 ounce) package frozen riced cauliflower

4 teaspoons olive oil

1 teaspoon no-salt-added taco seasoning

1 cup thinly sliced red cabbage

1 cup diced avocado

½ cup pico de gallo or salsa

¼ cup chopped fresh cilantro

How to Make

Prepare Tofu Crumbles as directed.

While the Tofu Crumbles cook, prepare riced cauliflower according to package directions. Toss with oil and taco seasoning.

Divide the cauliflower among 4 single-serving containers with lids. Top each with 1/2 cup Beefless Ground Beef, 1/4 cup each cabbage and avocado, 2 tablespoons pico de gallo (or salsa) and 1 tablespoon cilantro. Seal the containers and refrigerate until ready to eat.

Avocado Tuna Salad

Ingredients You Need

3 tablespoons extra-virgin olive oil

2 tablespoons lemon juice

¼ teaspoon salt

2 medium avocados, chopped (about 2 1/2 cups)

2 (5 ounce) cans solid white tuna in oil, drained and flaked

4 cups romaine hearts

1 cup chopped English cucumber

⅓ cup crumbled feta cheese

¼ cup toasted sliced almonds

¼ cup chopped pitted Kalamata olives

3 tablespoons chopped fresh flat-leaf parsley

How to Make

Whisk oil, lemon juice and salt together in a large bowl; add avocados and toss gently to coat thoroughly. Add tuna, romaine, cucumber, feta, almonds, olives and parsley to the avocado mixture; toss gently to combine. Serve immediately or refrigerate for up to 1 hour.

Chicken & Bok Choy Soup with Ginger & Mushrooms

Ingredients You Need

1/2 ounce (about 1/2 cup) dried shiitake or mixed dried mushrooms

3 cups boiling water

1 tablespoon peanut oil or canola oil

2 cups diced onion

3 cloves garlic, thinly sliced

6 1/8-inch-thick slices peeled fresh ginger

6 cups reduced-sodium chicken broth

¼ cup reduced-sodium soy sauce

1 2-to-3-inch cinnamon stick

1 whole star anise

1 teaspoon freshly ground pepper

2 pounds boneless, skinless chicken thighs, trimmed and cut into 1-inch pieces

1 bulb fennel, cored and cut into 1-inch pieces

8 scallions, whites cut into 2-inch pieces and greens chopped, divided

1 pound bok choy, preferably baby bok choy, white stems sliced lengthwise and greens chopped, divided

2 cups (4 ounces) mung bean sprouts (see Note)

½ cup chopped fresh cilantro

2 teaspoons toasted sesame oil

Lime wedges for garnish

How to Make

Place mushrooms in a heatproof measuring cup and cover with boiling water. Soak for at least 30 minutes or up to several hours. Remove the mushrooms from the water, remove and discard stems (if any) and cut into 1/8-inch slices; set aside. Strain the soaking liquid and reserve.

Heat oil in a large soup pot or Dutch oven over medium heat. Add onion, garlic and ginger and cook, stirring, for 5 minutes. Pour in the reserved mushroom liquid, broth, soy sauce, cinnamon stick, star anise and pepper. Bring to a boil. Reduce to a simmer and stir in chicken. Simmer for 20 minutes.

Stir in fennel, scallion whites and the reserved mushrooms and cook for 5 minutes. Add bok choy stems, return to a simmer and cook for 3 minutes more. Stir in bok choy greens and bean sprouts. Cook until the greens are just wilted, about 2 minutes more.

Discard the cinnamon stick and star anise. Ladle the soup into bowls. Garnish each bowl with scallion greens, cilantro and a 1/4-teaspoon drizzle of sesame oil. Serve with lime wedges, if desired.

What You Need

Large soup pot or Dutch oven

Zucchini Frittata

Ingredients You Need

4 teaspoons extra-virgin olive oil, divided

1 cup diced zucchini, (1 small)

½ cup chopped onion

1/2 cup grape tomatoes, or cherry tomatoes, halved

¼ cup slivered fresh mint

¼ cup slivered fresh basil

¼ teaspoon salt, divided

5 large eggs

Freshly ground pepper, to taste

1/3 cup crumbled goat cheese, (2 ounces)

How to Make

Heat 2 teaspoons oil in a 10-inch nonstick skillet over medium heat. Add zucchini and onion; cook, stirring often, for 1 minute. Cover and reduce heat to medium-low; cook, stirring occasionally, until the zucchini is tender, but not mushy, 3 to 5 minutes. Add tomatoes, mint, basil, 1/8 teaspoon salt and a grinding of pepper; increase heat to medium-high and cook, stirring, until the moisture has evaporated, 30 to 60 seconds.

Whisk eggs, the remaining 1/8 teaspoon salt and a grinding of pepper in a large bowl until blended. Add the zucchini mixture and cheese; stir to combine.

Preheat the broiler.

Wipe out the pan and brush it with the remaining 2 teaspoons oil; place over medium-low heat. Add the frittata mixture and cook, without stirring, until the bottom is light golden, 2 to 4 minutes. As it cooks, lift the edges and tilt the pan so uncooked egg will flow to the edges.

Place the pan under the broiler and broil until the frittata is set and the top is golden, 1 1/2 to 2 1/2 minutes. Loosen the edges and slide onto a plate. Cut into wedges and serve.

What You Need

10-inch nonstick skillet

Creamy Pesto Chicken Salad with Greens

Ingredients You Need

1 pound boneless, skinless chicken breast, trimmed

¼ cup pesto

¼ cup low-fat mayonnaise

3 tablespoons finely chopped red onion

2 tablespoons extra-virgin olive oil

2 tablespoons red-wine vinegar

¼ teaspoon salt

¼ teaspoon ground pepper

1 5-ounce package mixed salad greens (about 8 cups)

1 pint grape or cherry tomatoes, halved

How to Make

Place chicken in a medium saucepan and add water to cover by 1 inch. Bring to a boil. Cover, reduce heat to low and simmer gently until no longer pink in the middle, 10 to 15 minutes. Transfer to a clean cutting board; shred into bite-size pieces when cool enough to handle.

Combine pesto, mayonnaise and onion in a medium bowl. Add the chicken and toss to coat. Whisk oil, vinegar, salt and pepper in a large bowl. Add greens and tomatoes and toss to coat. Divide the green salad among 4 plates and top with the chicken salad.

Taco Lettuce Wraps

Ingredients You Need

8 small iceberg or romaine lettuce leaves or 4 large,
cut in half crosswise

1 tablespoon canola oil

1 pound lean ground beef

¼ teaspoon salt

5 tablespoons prepared salsa

1 tablespoon rice vinegar

1 ½ teaspoons ground cumin

1 cup diced avocado

1 cup julienned jícama (see Tip)

¼ cup finely diced red onion

How to Make

Wash and dry lettuce leaves well and cut out any tough ribs.

Heat oil in a large nonstick skillet over medium-high heat. Add ground beef, season with salt and cook, stirring often, until cooked through, 4 to 6 minutes.

Meanwhile, whisk salsa, vinegar and cumin in a small bowl.

Remove the pan from the heat, add the salsa mixture and stir to combine. Serve in the lettuce leaves, topped with avocado, jicama and onion.

Please Note

Jícama is a round root vegetable with thin brown skin and white crunchy flesh. It has a slightly sweet and nutty flavor. To peel it, use a small, sharp knife or vegetable peeler, making sure to remove both the papery brown skin and the layer of fibrous flesh just underneath.

Turkey & Cheddar Lettuce Wraps

Ingredients You Need

¼ cup mayonnaise

3 tablespoons chopped dill pickle

2 teaspoons whole-grain mustard

8 large green-leaf lettuce leaves

12 ounces sliced deli turkey

4 ounces sliced deli sharp Cheddar cheese

8 slices tomato

How to Make

Stir mayonnaise, pickle and mustard together in a small bowl.

Overlap 2 lettuce leaves on a clean cutting board. Spread a generous 1 tablespoon of the mayonnaise mixture over the lettuce. Top with 3 ounces turkey, 1 ounce cheese and 2 tomato slices. Roll into a wrap, then cut in half. Repeat with the remaining **Ingredients You Need.**

Arugula, Chicken & Melon Salad with Sumac

Ingredients You Need

¼ cup lemon juice

1 teaspoon ground sumac (see Tip), plus more for garnish

1 teaspoon honey

1 clove garlic, grated

¼ teaspoon salt

¼ cup extra-virgin olive oil

5 ounces baby arugula (8 cups)

2 cups shredded cooked chicken breast (about 12 ounces)

2 cups cantaloupe balls (from 1 small melon)

4 ounces feta cheese, preferably sheep's-milk, crumbled

1 cup fresh mint leaves, torn

¼ cup pine nuts, toasted

How to Make

Whisk lemon juice, sumac, honey, garlic and salt in a large bowl. Gradually whisk in oil until combined. Add arugula, chicken, melon, feta and mint. Toss to coat with the dressing. Sprinkle with pine nuts and garnish with additional sumac, if desired.

What You Need

Melon baller

Please Note

Sumac comes from the tart red berries of the Mediterranean sumac bush. It adds sour, fruity flavor and a pop of color to this dressing. Find it in the spice section of well-stocked grocery stores or online.

Chopped Power Salad with Chicken

Ingredients You Need

¼ cup extra-virgin olive oil

3 tablespoons lemon juice

1 clove garlic, grated

½ teaspoon dried oregano

½ teaspoon sugar

¼ teaspoon salt

¼ teaspoon ground pepper

4 cups torn green-leaf lettuce

4 cups baby spinach

2 cups shredded cooked chicken

1 cup halved grape tomatoes

1 cup halved and sliced cucumber

½ cup slivered red onion

⅓ cup sliced pepperoncini

⅓ cup crumbled feta cheese

2 tablespoons toasted unsalted sunflower seeds

How to Make

Whisk oil, lemon juice, garlic, oregano, sugar, salt and pepper together in a large bowl.

Add lettuce, spinach, chicken, tomatoes, cucumber, onion and pepperoncini; toss to coat. Serve sprinkled with feta and sunflower seeds.

Avocado Ranch Chicken Salad

Ingredients You Need

1 ripe avocado, halved and pitted

⅓ cup ranch dressing

2 tablespoons chopped pickled jalapeño

1 tablespoon white-wine vinegar

¼ teaspoon salt

¼ teaspoon ground pepper

3 cups shredded or chopped cooked chicken

½ cup diced celery

¼ cup diced red onion

How to Make

Scoop avocado into a food processor. Add ranch dressing, pickled jalapeño, vinegar, salt and pepper. Pulse until smooth. Transfer to a medium bowl. Add chicken, celery and red onion; mix with a rubber spatula. Serve at room temperature or refrigerate until cold, about 2 hours.

Please Note

To make ahead: Refrigerate, covered, for up to 1 day.

Salmon-Stuffed Avocados

Ingredients You Need

½ cup nonfat plain Greek yogurt

½ cup diced celery

2 tablespoons chopped fresh parsley

1 tablespoon lime juice

2 teaspoons mayonnaise

1 teaspoon Dijon mustard

⅛ teaspoon salt

⅛ teaspoon ground pepper

2 (5 ounce) cans salmon, drained, flaked, skin and bones removed

2 avocados

Chopped chives for garnish

How to Make

Combine yogurt, celery, parsley, lime juice, mayonnaise, mustard, salt, and pepper in a medium bowl; mix well. Add salmon and mix well.

Halve avocados lengthwise and remove pits. Scoop about 1 tablespoon flesh from each avocado half into a small bowl. Mash the scooped-out avocado flesh with a fork and stir into the salmon mixture.

Fill each avocado half with about 1/4 cup of the salmon mixture, mounding it on top of the avocado halves. Garnish with chives, if desired.

Chopped Salad with Sriracha Tofu

Ingredients You Need

1 (10 ounce) package kale, Brussels sprout, broccoli and cabbage salad mix

1 (12 ounce) package frozen shelled edamame, thawed

2 (7 ounce) packages Sriracha-flavored baked tofu, cubed

1/2 cup spicy peanut vinaigrette

How to Make

Divide salad mix among 4 single-serving containers with lids. Top each with 1/2 cup edamame and one-fourth of the tofu.

Transfer 2 tablespoons vinaigrette into each of 4 small lidded containers and refrigerate for up to 4 days.

Seal the salad containers and refrigerate for up to 4 days. Dress with vinaigrette up to 1 day before serving.

Please Note

To make ahead: Refrigerate for up to 4 days.

CHAPTER 7
HIGH PROTEIN, LOW-CALORIE LUNCH
RECIPES

Roasted Red Pepper Stuffed Chicken Breast

Ingredients You Need

½ cup crumbled feta cheese

½ cup chopped roasted red bell peppers

½ cup chopped fresh spinach

¼ cup Kalamata olives, pitted and quartered

1 tablespoon chopped fresh basil

1 tablespoon chopped fresh flat-leaf parsley

2 cloves garlic, minced

4 (8 ounce) boneless, skinless chicken breasts

¼ teaspoon salt

½ teaspoon ground pepper

1 tablespoon extra-virgin olive oil

1 tablespoon lemon juice

How to Make

Preheat oven to 400°F. Combine feta, roasted red peppers, spinach, olives, basil, parsley and garlic in a medium bowl.

Using a small knife, cut a horizontal slit through the thickest portion of each chicken breast to form a pocket. Stuff each breast pocket with about 1/3 cup of the feta mixture; secure the pockets using wooden picks. Sprinkle the chicken evenly with salt and pepper.

Heat oil in a large oven-safe skillet over medium-high heat. Arrange the stuffed breasts, top-sides down, in the pan; cook until golden, about 2 minutes. Carefully flip the chicken; transfer the pan to the oven. Bake until an instant-read thermometer inserted in the thickest portion of the chicken registers 165°F, 20 to 25 minutes. Drizzle the chicken evenly with lemon juice. Remove the wooden picks from the chicken before serving.

Chicken Cutlets with Creamy Pesto Sauce

Ingredients You Need

1 pound chicken cutlets

¼ teaspoon salt, divided

¼ teaspoon ground pepper, divided

1 tablespoon extra-virgin olive oil

½ cup finely chopped red onion

½ cup dry white wine

½ cup heavy cream

¼ cup pesto

1 medium plum tomato, chopped

2 tablespoons chopped basil

How to Make

Sprinkle chicken with 1/8 teaspoon salt and 1/8 teaspoon pepper. Heat oil in a large skillet over medium-high heat. Add the chicken and cook, turning once, until browned and cooked through, about 6 minutes. Transfer to a plate.

Add onion to the pan. Cook, stirring, for 1 minute. Increase heat to high and add wine. Cook, scraping up any browned bits, until the liquid is mostly evaporated, about 2 minutes. Reduce heat to medium and stir in cream, any accumulated juices from the chicken and the remaining 1/8 teaspoon each salt and pepper; simmer for 2 minutes. Stir in pesto and tomatoes, then return the chicken to the pan. Turn to coat; cook until warmed through, about 1 minute. Divide the chicken and sauce among 4 plates. Sprinkle with basil.

Chicken & Mushrooms

Ingredients You Need

4 4- to 5-ounce chicken cutlets (see Tips)

4 cups mixed mushrooms, sliced if large

½ cup dry white wine

½ cup heavy cream

2 tablespoons finely chopped fresh parsley

How to Make

Sprinkle chicken with 1/4 teaspoon each kosher salt and pepper. Heat 1 tablespoon canola oil in a large skillet over medium heat. Cook the chicken, turning once, until browned and just cooked through, 7 to 10 minutes total. Transfer to a plate.

Add 1 tablespoon oil and mushrooms to the pan; cook, stirring occasionally, until the liquid has evaporated, about 4 minutes. Increase heat to high, add wine and cook until it has mostly evaporated, about 4 minutes. Reduce heat to medium; stir in cream, any accumulated juice from the chicken and 1/4 teaspoon each salt and pepper. Return the chicken to the pan and turn to coat with the sauce. Serve the chicken topped with the sauce and sprinkled with parsley.

Poulet au Vinaigre

Ingredients You Need

1 ¼ pounds boneless, skinless chicken thighs, trimmed

½ teaspoon salt plus a pinch, divided

¼ teaspoon ground pepper

¼ cup all-purpose flour

2 tablespoons unsalted butter

2 tablespoons grapeseed or canola oil

4 cloves garlic, sliced

1 large shallot, sliced

1 tablespoon tomato paste

1 large tomato, seeded and diced

¼ cup red-wine vinegar

1 tablespoon honey

1 ½ cups low-sodium chicken broth

1 tablespoon chopped fresh parsley

1 tablespoon chopped fresh tarragon

How to Make

Pat chicken dry and season with 1/2 teaspoon salt
and pepper. Place flour in a shallow bowl and toss

the chicken in it to coat, shaking off excess. (Discard the remaining flour.)

Heat butter and oil in a large skillet over medium-high heat until foamy. Add the chicken and cook, flipping once, until brown on both sides, 9 to 12 minutes total. Add garlic, shallot and the remaining pinch of salt; cook for 1 minute. Add tomato paste; cook for 1 minute. Stir in tomato, vinegar and honey, scraping up any browned bits. Stir in broth. Bring to a simmer.

Reduce heat to low, cover and cook for 15 minutes. Uncover and cook, flipping the chicken occasionally, until the sauce is slightly thickened, 20 to 25 minutes more. Stir in parsley and tarragon.

Salmon & Asparagus with Lemon-Garlic Butter Sauce

Ingredients You Need

1 pound center-cut salmon fillet, preferably wild, cut into 4 portions

1 pound fresh asparagus, trimmed

½ teaspoon salt

½ teaspoon ground pepper

3 tablespoons butter

1 tablespoon extra-virgin olive oil

½ tablespoon grated garlic

1 teaspoon grated lemon zest

1 tablespoon lemon juice

How to Make

Preheat oven to 375 degrees F. Coat a large rimmed baking sheet with cooking spray.

Place salmon on one side of the prepared baking sheet and asparagus on the other. Sprinkle the salmon and asparagus with salt and pepper.

Heat butter, oil, garlic, lemon zest and lemon juice in a small skillet over medium heat until the butter is melted. Drizzle the butter mixture over the salmon and asparagus. Bake until the salmon is cooked through and the asparagus is just tender, 12 to 15 minutes.

Skillet Lemon Chicken with Spinach

Ingredients You Need

2 tablespoons extra-virgin olive oil

1 pound boneless, skinless chicken thighs, trimmed and cut into bite-size pieces

1 cup diced red bell pepper

½ teaspoon salt

½ teaspoon ground pepper

4 cloves garlic, minced

½ cup dry white wine

1 teaspoon cornstarch

1 medium lemon, zested and juiced

10 cups lightly packed baby spinach

8 teaspoons grated Parmesan cheese

How to Make

Heat oil in a large skillet over medium-high heat. Add chicken, bell pepper, salt and pepper; cook, stirring occasionally, until the chicken is just cooked through, 7 to 9 minutes. Add garlic and cook, stirring, until fragrant, about 1 minute. Whisk wine and cornstarch together in a measuring cup. Add to the pan along with the lemon juice and zest; stir to coat, then bring to a simmer. Add spinach by the handful; cook, stirring, until wilted, about 2 minutes more. Serve sprinkled with Parmesan.

Coriander-&-Lemon-Crusted Salmon with Asparagus Salad & Poached Egg

Ingredients You Need

1 tablespoon coriander seeds

1 teaspoon lemon zest

¾ teaspoon fine sea salt, divided

½ teaspoon crushed red pepper

1 pound wild salmon (see Tips), skin-on, cut into 4 portions

1 pound asparagus, trimmed

2 tablespoons extra-virgin olive oil

1 tablespoon lemon juice

1 tablespoon chopped fresh mint

1 tablespoon chopped fresh tarragon

¼ teaspoon ground pepper, plus more for garnish

8 cups water

1 tablespoon white vinegar

4 large eggs

How to Make

Position a rack in upper third of oven; preheat broiler to high. Coat a rimmed baking sheet with cooking spray.

Toast coriander in a small skillet over medium heat, shaking the pan frequently, until fragrant, about 3 minutes. Pulse the coriander, lemon zest, 1/2 teaspoon salt and crushed red pepper in a spice grinder until finely ground. Coat the salmon flesh with the spice mixture (about 1 1/2 teaspoons per portion) and place the salmon on the prepared baking sheet.

Cut off asparagus tips and very thinly slice stalks on the diagonal. Toss the tips and slices with oil, lemon juice, mint, tarragon, pepper and the remaining 1/4 teaspoon salt. Let stand while you cook the salmon and eggs.

Bring water and vinegar to a boil in a large saucepan.

Meanwhile, broil the salmon until just cooked through, 3 to 6 minutes, depending on thickness (see Tips). Tent with foil to keep warm.

Reduce the boiling water to a bare simmer. Gently stir in a circle so the water is swirling around the pot. Crack eggs, one at a time, into the water. Cook until the whites are set but the yolks are still runny, 3 to 4 minutes.

To serve, divide the asparagus salad and salmon among 4 plates. Make a nest in each salad and top with a poached egg.

Chicken with Lemon-Caper Pan Sauce

Ingredients You Need

2 8-ounce boneless, skinless chicken breasts

½ teaspoon salt, divided

½ teaspoon ground pepper, divided

¼ cup white whole-wheat flour

3 tablespoons extra-virgin olive oil, divided

½ cup thinly sliced leek

2 tablespoons sliced shallot

1 tablespoon lemon zest

¼ cup lemon juice

1 cup low-sodium chicken broth

1 tablespoon capers

1 tablespoon butter

How to Make

Remove and reserve chicken tenders (if attached) for another use. Slice each breast in half horizontally to make 4 pieces total. Place on a cutting board and cover with a large piece of plastic wrap. Pound with the smooth side of a meat mallet or a heavy saucepan to an even thickness of about 1/4 inch. Sprinkle with 1/4 teaspoon each salt and pepper. Place flour in a shallow dish and dredge the cutlets to coat both sides, shaking off excess. (Discard remaining flour.)

Heat 2 tablespoons oil in a large skillet over medium-high heat. Add 2 pieces of chicken and cook, turning once, until evenly browned and cooked through, 2 to 3 minutes per side. Transfer to a large serving plate and tent with foil to keep warm. Repeat with the remaining chicken.

Add the remaining 1 tablespoon oil, leek and shallot to the pan. Cook, stirring occasionally, until just softened, 1 to 2 minutes. Add lemon juice; bring to a boil. Cook, scraping up any browned bits from the bottom of the pan, until the lemon juice is reduced by about half, about 45 seconds. Add broth, zest, capers and the remaining 1/4 teaspoon salt and pepper. Cook, stirring, until the sauce is reduced by about half, 4 to 7 minutes.

Remove from heat; stir in butter. Serve the sauce over the chicken.

Frittata with Asparagus, Leek & Ricotta

Ingredients You Need

8 large eggs

¼ cup crème fraîche

½ teaspoon salt

¼ teaspoon ground pepper

2 tablespoons extra-virgin olive oil

3 cups thinly sliced leeks (about 2 medium), rinsed well and patted dry

1 pound asparagus, trimmed and cut into 1-inch pieces

¼ cup part-skim ricotta

2 tablespoons pesto

¼ cup fresh basil

How to Make

Position rack in upper third of oven; preheat broiler.

Whisk eggs, crème fraîche, salt and pepper in a medium bowl; set near the stove. Heat oil in a large cast-iron skillet over medium-high heat. Add leeks and asparagus and cook, stirring frequently, until soft, 5 to 6 minutes.

Pour the egg mixture over the vegetables and cook, lifting the edges so uncooked egg can flow underneath, until nearly set, about 2 minutes. Dollop ricotta and pesto on top and place the pan under the broiler until the eggs are slightly browned, 1 1/2 to 2 minutes. Let stand for 3 minutes.

Run a spatula around the edge of the frittata, then underneath, until you can slide or lift it out onto a cutting board or serving plate. Top with basil.

Meyer Lemon Chicken Piccata

Ingredients You Need

2 (8-ounce) skinless, boneless chicken breast halves

½ teaspoon kosher salt

¼ teaspoon freshly ground black pepper

¼ cup all-purpose flour

2 tablespoons unsalted butter, divided

⅓ cup sauvignon blanc or other crisp, tart white wine

½ cup fat-free, lower-sodium chicken broth

⅓ cup fresh Meyer lemon juice (about 3 lemons)

2 tablespoons capers, rinsed and drained

¼ cup chopped fresh flat-leaf parsley

How to Make

Split chicken breast halves in half horizontally to form 4 cutlets. Place each cutlet between 2 sheets of heavy-duty plastic wrap; pound each cutlet to 1/4-inch thickness using a meat mallet or small heavy skillet. Sprinkle cutlets evenly with salt and pepper. Place flour in a shallow dish; dredge cutlets in flour.

Melt 1 tablespoon butter in a large skillet over medium-high heat. Add 2 cutlets to pan, and sauté 2 minutes. Turn cutlets over; sauté for 1 minute. Remove the cutlets from pan. Repeat the procedure with remaining 1 tablespoon butter and 2 cutlets.

Add wine to pan, and bring to a boil, scraping pan to loosen browned bits. Cook for 1 minute or until liquid almost evaporates. Stir in chicken broth; bring to a boil. Cook until broth mixture is reduced to 2 tablespoons (about 4 minutes). Stir in juice and capers. Serve over chicken. Sprinkle with parsley.

Pesto Shrimp

Ingredients You Need

2 tablespoons extra-virgin olive oil, divided

1 ½ pounds large peeled, deveined raw shrimp

1 teaspoon no-salt-added Italian seasoning

1 pint grape tomatoes

2 cups loosely packed fresh basil leaves

½ cup refrigerated basil pesto

How to Make

Heat 1 tablespoon oil in a large nonstick skillet over medium-high heat. Add shrimp and Italian seasoning; cook, stirring often, until the shrimp are just cooked through and turn opaque, 3 to 5 minutes. Transfer the shrimp to a plate. Wipe the pan clean.

Add the remaining 1 tablespoon oil to the pan; heat over medium heat. Add tomatoes; cook, stirring occasionally and pressing the tomatoes down lightly with tongs or a wooden spoon, until the tomatoes begin to break down and juices are released, about 5 minutes. Add basil and return the shrimp to the pan. Cook, stirring constantly, until the basil is wilted and the shrimp are warm, about 1 minute. Remove from heat; stir in pesto.

Sautéed Striped Bass with Lemon

Ingredients You Need

4 (5 ounce) skin-on striped bass fillets (either hybrid striped bass or wild), patted dry

¼ teaspoon black pepper

1 teaspoon kosher salt, divided

1 lemon, halved lengthwise

3 tablespoons olive oil

2 tablespoons dry white wine

2 tablespoons cold unsalted butter

2 tablespoons chopped fresh parsley

How to Make

Sprinkle fillets with pepper and 3/4 teaspoon salt; let stand 20 minutes.

Heat a large nonstick skillet over medium-high. Add lemons, cut sides down, and cook until lightly charred, about 5 minutes. Add olive oil, and place fillets, skin sides down, in skillet with lemon. Cook, undisturbed, until sides of skin begin to brown and fish is almost fully opaque, 5 to 7 minutes.

When the fillets appear to be approximately 90% cooked through, gently shake skillet. When cooked with patience, the fish will release itself from the pan, allowing you to flip the fillets without sticking. Flip fillets, and cook 1 minute. Transfer fish and lemons to plates. Cut each lemon half into 2 wedges. Wipe skillet clean.

Reduce heat to medium-low, and add wine, remaining 1/4 teaspoon salt and butter. As butter melts, whisk to emulsify mixture. Spoon sauce over fillets. Sprinkle with parsley, and serve with a charred lemon wedge

Pistachio-Crusted Halibut

Ingredients You Need

1 ¼ pounds halibut, cut into 4 portions

½ teaspoon kosher salt

¼ teaspoon ground pepper

1 tablespoon reduced-fat mayonnaise

3 tablespoons chopped unsalted pistachios

3 tablespoons panko breadcrumbs

1 large clove garlic, grated

How to Make

Preheat oven to 425°F. Coat a baking sheet with cooking spray.

Pat halibut fillets dry with paper towels and place on the prepared pan. Sprinkle with salt and pepper. Brush the tops of the fillets with mayonnaise. Combine pistachios, panko and garlic in a small bowl. Top the fillets with the pistachio mixture, gently pressing to adhere.

Bake until the fish flakes easily with a fork, 8 to 12 minutes, depending on the thickness.

Grilled Salmon & Vegetables

Ingredients You Need

2 medium zucchini, trimmed and halved lengthwise

1 pound asparagus, trimmed

5 - 6 tablespoons Charred Lemon-Garlic Vinaigrette, divided

1 ¼ pounds salmon fillet, cut into 4 portions

¼ teaspoon salt, divided

¼ teaspoon ground pepper, divided

How to Make

Preheat grill to medium-high.

Brush zucchini and asparagus with 2 tablespoons vinaigrette and sprinkle with 1/8 teaspoon each salt and pepper. Drizzle salmon with 2 teaspoons vinaigrette and sprinkle with the remaining 1/8 teaspoon each salt and pepper.

Place the vegetables and the salmon pieces, skin-side down, on the grill. Grill the vegetables, turning a few times, until tender, 6 to 8 minutes. Grill the salmon, without turning, until it flakes with a fork, 8 to 10 minutes.

Cut the vegetables into 3 or 4 pieces and place in a medium bowl. Drizzle with 2 tablespoons vinaigrette and toss to coat. Remove the skin from the salmon, if desired; serve the salmon alongside the vegetables. Drizzle the salmon with 1 tablespoon vinaigrette, if desired. (Refrigerate any remaining vinaigrette for up to 3 days.)

Grilled Bone-In Pork Chops

Ingredients You Need

1 cup water

¼ cup honey

1 tablespoon apple cider vinegar

½ teaspoon crushed red pepper

4 ½ teaspoons kosher salt, divided

4 (6 ounce) bone-in, center-cut pork chops (about 1-inch thick)

1 tablespoon olive oil

1 teaspoon black pepper

How to Make

Stir together water, honey, vinegar, crushed red pepper and 4 teaspoons of the salt in a small bowl until honey and salt are dissolved. Place pork chops and water mixture in a zip-top plastic bag; seal and refrigerate 1 hour.

Preheat a grill or grill pan to high (450°F to 500°F). Remove chops from bag; discard marinade and pat chops very dry with paper towels. Drizzle chops evenly with oil on both sides; sprinkle with black pepper and remaining 1/2 teaspoon salt.

Place chops on oiled grates; grill, covered, until a thermometer inserted in the thickest portion of meat registers 140°F, about 4 minutes per side. Remove from grill; let rest 5 minutes.

Cheesy Portobello Chicken Cutlets with Broccoli

Ingredients You Need

2 tablespoons extra-virgin olive oil, divided

4 chicken cutlets (about 1 pound)

½ teaspoon salt, divided

½ teaspoon ground pepper, divided

1 large head broccoli, cut into 2- to 3-inch spears

¼ cup water

1 cup sliced onion

1 large portobello mushroom cap, stem and gills removed, sliced

2 tablespoons balsamic vinegar

2 tablespoons Worcestershire sauce

1 teaspoon Dijon mustard

2 tablespoons chopped fresh thyme, plus more for garnish

4 ounces sliced Gruyère cheese

Chopped fresh parsley for garnish

How to Make

Heat 1 tablespoon oil in a large broiler-safe skillet over medium-high heat. Season chicken with 1/4 teaspoon each salt and pepper and add to the pan. Cook, flipping once, until golden and an instant-read thermometer inserted in the thickest part registers 165°F, about 6 minutes. Transfer to a plate.

Reduce heat to medium. Add 2 teaspoons oil and broccoli to the pan. Cook, stirring occasionally, until browned, about 5 minutes. Add water, cover and cook until tender, about 5 minutes more. Transfer to the plate with the chicken.

Add the remaining 1 teaspoon oil, onion and mushroom to the pan. Cook, stirring occasionally, until lightly browned, 5 to 8 minutes. Stir in vinegar, Worcestershire, mustard, thyme, the remaining 1/4 teaspoon each salt and pepper and any accumulated chicken juices from the plate. Cook, stirring and scraping up any browned bits, for 1 minute.

Meanwhile, position rack in upper third of oven; preheat broiler to high.

Return the chicken to the pan and spoon the mushroom mixture on top. Arrange the broccoli around the chicken. Top with cheese. Broil until the cheese is golden brown, 1 to 2 minutes. Serve topped with parsley and/or more thyme, if desired.

Air-Fryer Stuffed Chiles with Pork

Ingredients You Need

4 poblano peppers

Cooking spray

8 ounces lean ground pork

¾ cup diced zucchini

½ cup chopped white onion

½ cup rinsed canned black beans

1 tablespoon chili powder

½ teaspoon garlic powder

½ teaspoon salt

¼ teaspoon ground pepper

½ cup sour cream

¼ cup chopped fresh cilantro, plus more for garnish

½ cup crumbled cotija cheese

Tortilla chips & salsa verde for serving (optional)

How to Make

Lightly coat poblanos with cooking spray. Arrange in a single layer in the basket of a 6-quart air fryer. Cook at 400°F, flipping once, until the skins are charred, about 10 to 12 minutes. Transfer to a bowl, cover with plastic wrap and let steam for 10 minutes.

Meanwhile, cook pork, zucchini and onion in a large skillet over medium heat, stirring and breaking up the pork with a wooden spoon, until the pork is cooked through and the zucchini is tender, 5 to 8 minutes.

Add black beans, chili powder, garlic powder, salt and pepper; cook, stirring, for about 2 minutes. Remove from heat and stir in sour cream and cilantro.

Carefully peel the skin from the peppers and cut a slit, lengthwise, down one side of each pepper; remove and discard seeds.

Gently stuff the peppers with the pork mixture. Carefully arrange the peppers in the air-fryer basket (they'll be delicate). Cook at 400°F until heated through, about 5 minutes.

Top the stuffed chiles with cotija. Sprinkle with additional cilantro, if desired. Serve with chips and salsa, if desired.

What You Need

6-quart air fryer

Shrimp Cobb Salad with Dijon Dressing

Ingredients You Need

3 tablespoons extra-virgin olive oil

3 tablespoons white-wine vinegar

2 tablespoons finely chopped shallot

1 tablespoon Dijon mustard

½ teaspoon ground pepper

¼ teaspoon salt

10 cups mixed greens

12 cooked extra-large shrimp (16-20 count), peeled and halved lengthwise

1 cup halved cherry tomatoes

1 cup Persian cucumber chunks

2 large hard-boiled eggs, peeled and halved

1 avocado, diced

2 slices cooked bacon, crumbled

¼ cup crumbled blue cheese

How to Make

Place oil, vinegar, shallot, mustard, pepper and salt in a lidded jar. Shake until combined.

Mound salad greens on a platter. Drizzle with half the dressing and toss to coat. Decoratively arrange shrimp, tomatoes, cucumber, egg halves, avocado, bacon and blue cheese on top. Drizzle with the remaining dressing.

Mushroom Pork Chops

Ingredients You Need

4 (8 ounce) bone-in center-cut pork chops, about 3/4-inch thick

½ teaspoon salt

¾ teaspoon ground pepper, divided

3 tablespoons extra-virgin olive oil, divided

1 (5 ounce) package sliced fresh shiitake mushrooms

¼ cup thinly sliced shallot

4 cloves garlic, thinly sliced

½ cup dry sherry

1 (10.5 ounce) can low-sodium cream of mushroom soup

¾ cup water

1 teaspoon lower-sodium Worcestershire sauce

1 teaspoon Dijon mustard

1 tablespoon thinly sliced fresh chives

How to Make

Let pork chops stand at room temperature for 10 minutes. Pat dry with paper towels and sprinkle evenly with salt and 1/2 teaspoon pepper. Heat 2 tablespoons oil in a large cast-iron skillet over medium-high heat; add the pork chops and cook, undisturbed, until golden brown on 1 side, 4 to 5 minutes. Flip and cook for 1 minute more. Transfer the pork chops to a plate (they will not be cooked through); do not wipe the pan clean.

Add mushrooms to the pan; cook over medium-high heat, stirring occasionally, until golden brown, about 4 minutes. Add shallot, garlic and the remaining 1 tablespoon oil; cook, stirring occasionally, until the shallot is softened, about 3 minutes. Add sherry; cook, stirring constantly and scraping up browned bits from the bottom of the pan, until the liquid is almost completely reduced, about 1 minute. Add soup and water; cook, stirring, until the mixture comes to a simmer. Stir in Worcestershire, mustard and the remaining 1/4 teaspoon pepper.

Nestle the pork chops, browned-side up, into the mixture in the pan; cook over medium-high heat until an instant-read thermometer inserted in the thickest portion registers 145°F, about 8 minutes. Transfer the pork chops to 4 plates or a large platter; spoon the mushroom sauce over the chops. Sprinkle with chives.

Beef Stir-Fry with Baby Bok Choy & Ginger

Ingredients You Need

12 ounces beef flank steak, trimmed

1 tablespoon minced fresh ginger

1 ½ teaspoons reduced-sodium soy sauce

1 teaspoon dry sherry plus 1 Tbsp., divided

1 teaspoon cornstarch

1 teaspoon toasted sesame oil

2 tablespoons oyster-flavored sauce, preferably Lee Kum Kee Premium

1 tablespoon vegetable oil

1 pound baby bok choy, trimmed and cut into 2-inch pieces (about 8 cups)

3 tablespoons unsalted chicken broth

How to Make

Cut beef with the grain into 2-inch-wide strips. Cut each strip across the grain into 1/4-inch-thick slices. Combine the beef, ginger, soy sauce, 1 tsp. sherry, and cornstarch in a medium bowl; stir until the cornstarch is no longer visible. Add sesame oil and stir until the beef is lightly coated.

Combine oyster-flavored sauce and the remaining 1 Tbsp. sherry in a small bowl. Set aside.

Heat a 14-inch flat-bottomed carbon-steel wok (or a 12-inch stainless-steel skillet) over high heat until a drop of water vaporizes within 1 to 2 seconds of contact. Swirl in vegetable oil. Add the beef in an even layer; cook, undisturbed, until it begins to brown, about 1 minute. Using a metal spatula, stir-fry until lightly browned but not cooked through, 30 seconds to 1 minute more. Transfer to a plate.

Add bok choy and broth to the pan. Cover and cook until the bok choy greens are bright green and almost all the liquid has been absorbed, 1 to 2 minutes. Return the beef to the pan, add the reserved sauce, and stir-fry until the beef is just cooked through and the bok choy is tender-crisp, 30 seconds to 1 minute.

What You Need

14-inch flat-bottomed carbon-steel wok or 12-inch stainless-steel skillet